My Belly Has Two Buttons

Written By

Meikele Lee

Illustrated By

Rebecca Robertson

Layout and Formatting by Publishing Our Children's Stories,
Jesse Butler in 2016
First edition; First printing

Design and writing   © 2016 Meikele Needles

fb.me/meikele.lee
needlesmama2010@blogspot.com

Illustrations by Rebecca Robertson

Author Photo by Mary Williams of
queenelizabethphotography.com

ISBN 978-0-9984095-0-4

dedication

To my children, big things really do come in small packages and I hope

you never lose the strength to overcome whatever life throws your way.

I love you.

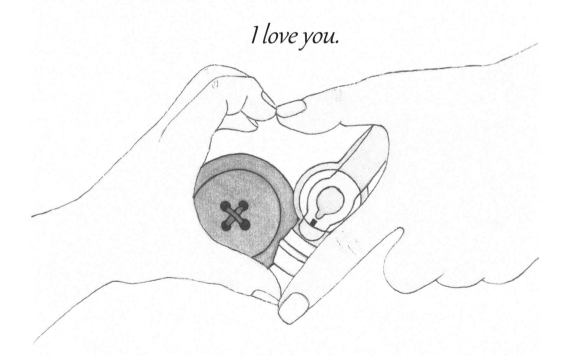

Hello, I am Nico. I am always Ready...Set...Go! I am like most 2-year-old boys you know.

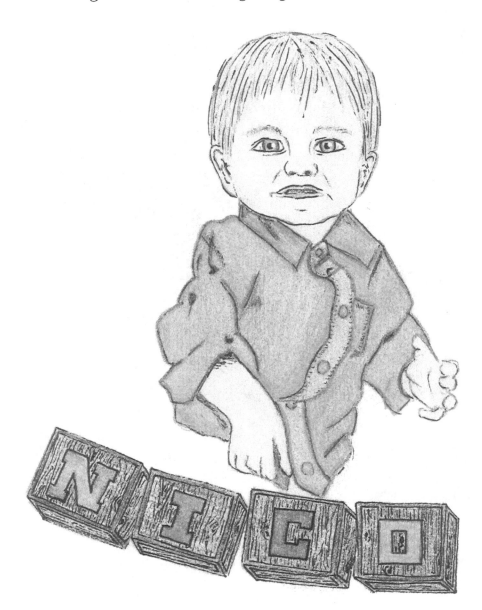

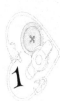

I love trains, blocks, and head buttin', but something special about me is, I have two buttons on my belly!

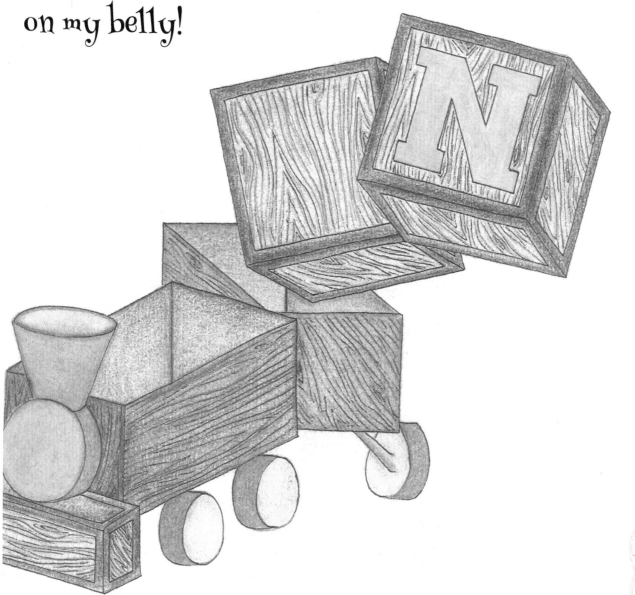

One is like everyone else's, the other is my Mic-key. My Mic-key is unique as you can see. I've only met two kids with 2 belly buttons like me.

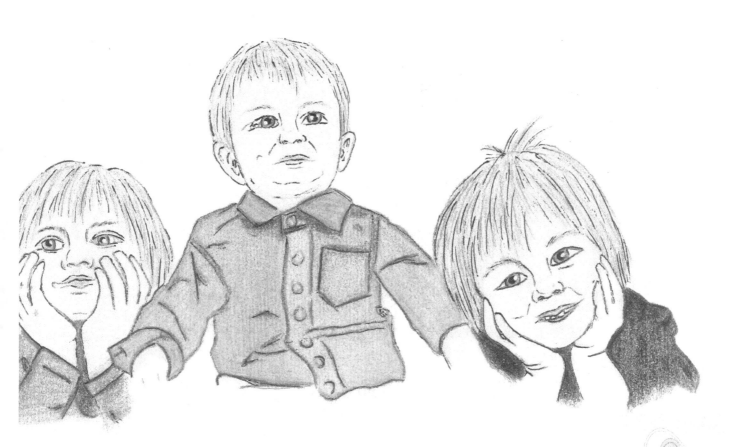

3

My Mic-Key is cool, it spins once a day, but my parents tell me, "keep your hands away," so, with it I cannot play.

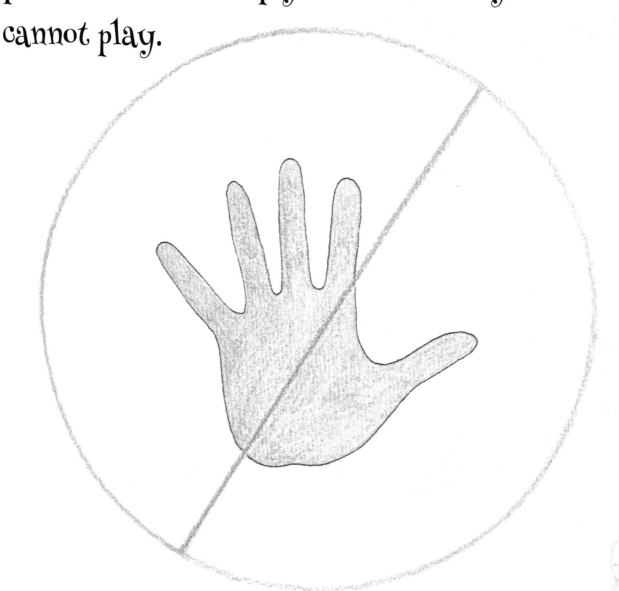

4

For a while, I was "NPO," which is Doctor's orders that nothing into my mouth could go.

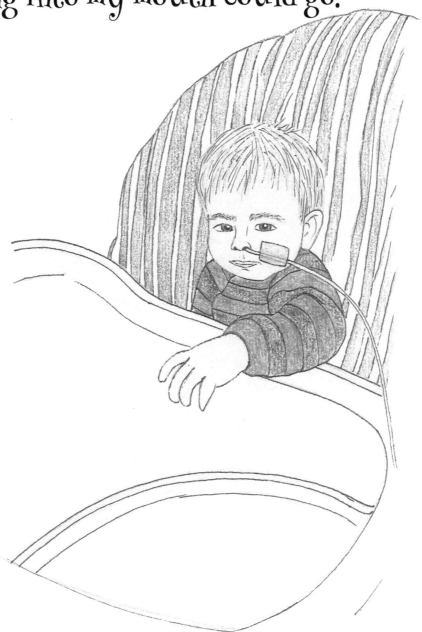

Medicine, water, and food that is what goes in my tube. They keep my body hydrated and fueled.

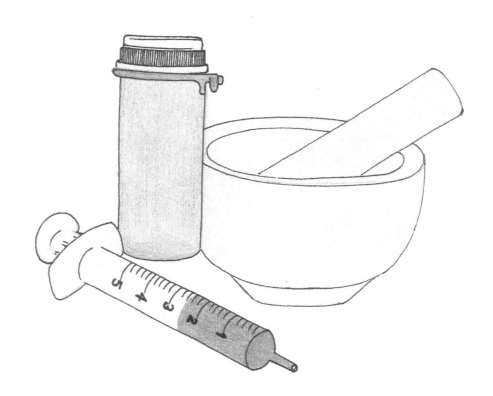

My Mic-Key opens and mom twists the tube. This happens because I need water, but can't safely consume.

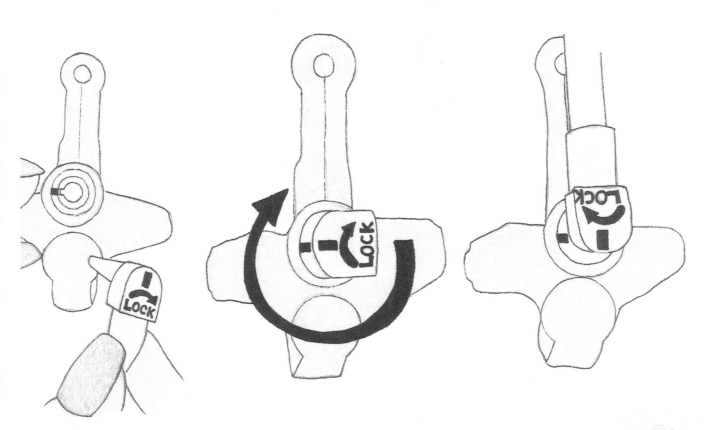

7

The Doctor's and Specialists aren't sure why, my body struggles to let me try. When I attempt I cough and choke.   Because of this, I drink like a slow   poke.

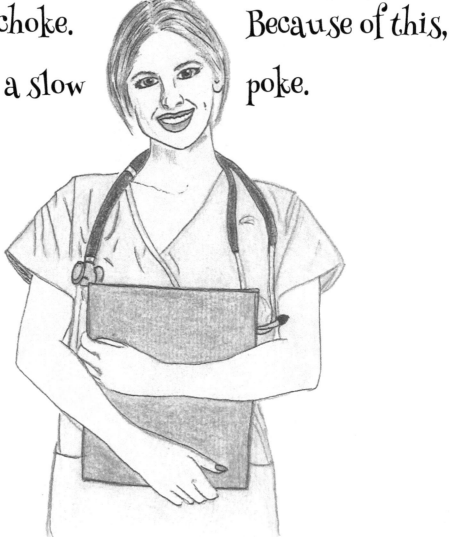

No bottles, straws or sippy cups, you'll see, not even when I was a baby. I am thankful for my therapists and parents who keep on tryin' to help me.

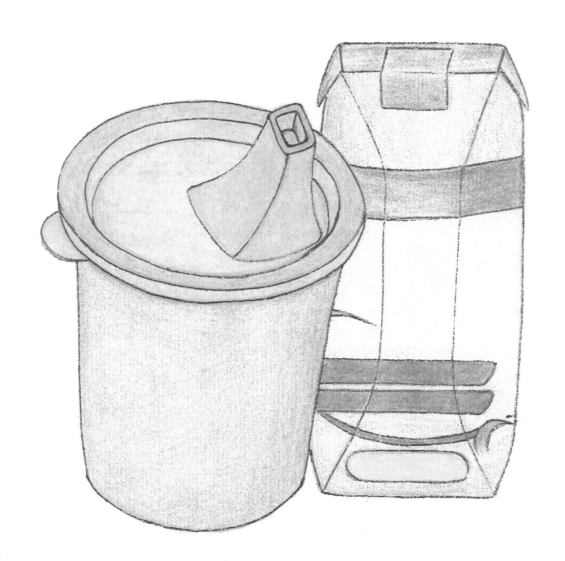

My feeding bag and tube hang from a pole. On it is a pump that keeps my tummy from being too full, but when I am attached you don't want to pull.

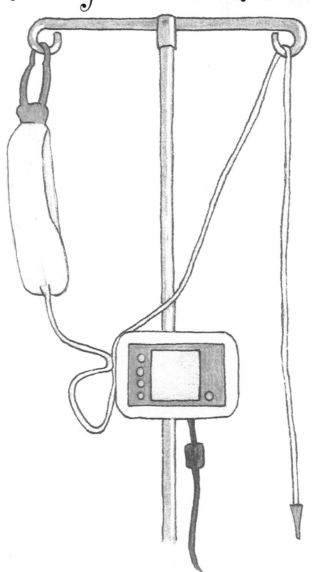

I am hooked up all night long, it helps me grow big and strong. Slowly, I am learning to eat new foods but like all 2-year-olds it depends on my moods.

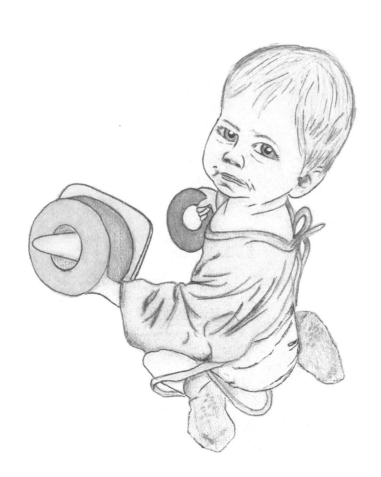

11

My Mic-key doesn't limit me. My doctor makes sure it fits my tummy. As I grow, it grows, but you never know because the peg never shows.

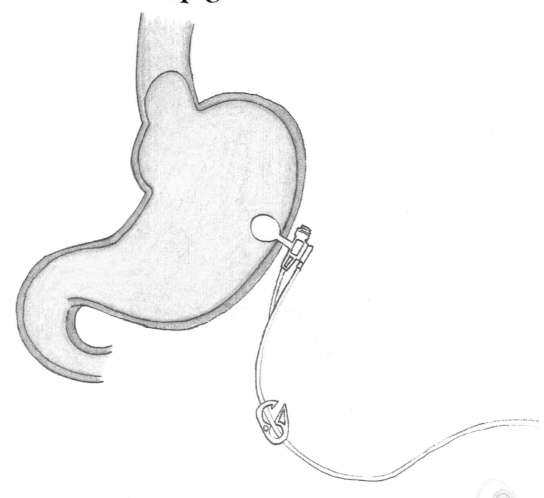

When I play, I have to be careful my button doesn't snag. It's held in my tummy by a water balloon, but don't worry, I can still play tag. My protective belt keeps it safe, but it's hot and can make my skin chafe.

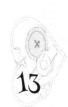

13

Please don't feel sorry for me, I might have it out by the time I am 3! But with me, you just have to wait and see. So until I graduate, I will love my two buttons, and not let it slow down my struttin'.

3

14

About the Author

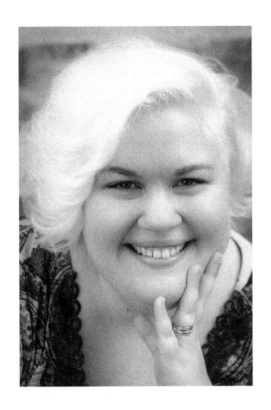

Meikele Lee is the author of the children's book "My Belly has Two Buttons" and lives in Helena, MT. She is a wife and mother to 3 amazing children, one of whom has a feeding tube. She has been in cosmetology for over 10 years, but became passionate about blogging when her youngest child's oral aversions became life threatening. She used blogging to try and understand her son's condition and how he can relate to others with or without a feeding tube. Blogging also helps to educate the public about these life saving devices. You can find her at needlesmama2010@blogspot.com

About the Illustrator

Rebecca Robertson born in Carthage, NY, now age 26 resides in Bellevue, WA with her husband Adam of 6 years. Since a young age she has always had a flair for creativity and a passion that led her to many artistic hobbies. Among these have been oil canvas' specialty painting's, Henna and now Illustration. She plans to continue along her very eclectic path and share her many talents in hopes to bring positivity, excitement, and genuine understanding of the unique and beautiful things in this world that can only be expressed through Art.

CPSIA information can be obtained
at www.ICGtesting.com
Printed in the USA
LVHW061416241119
638248LV00009B/182/P